SHTF Survival Pantry

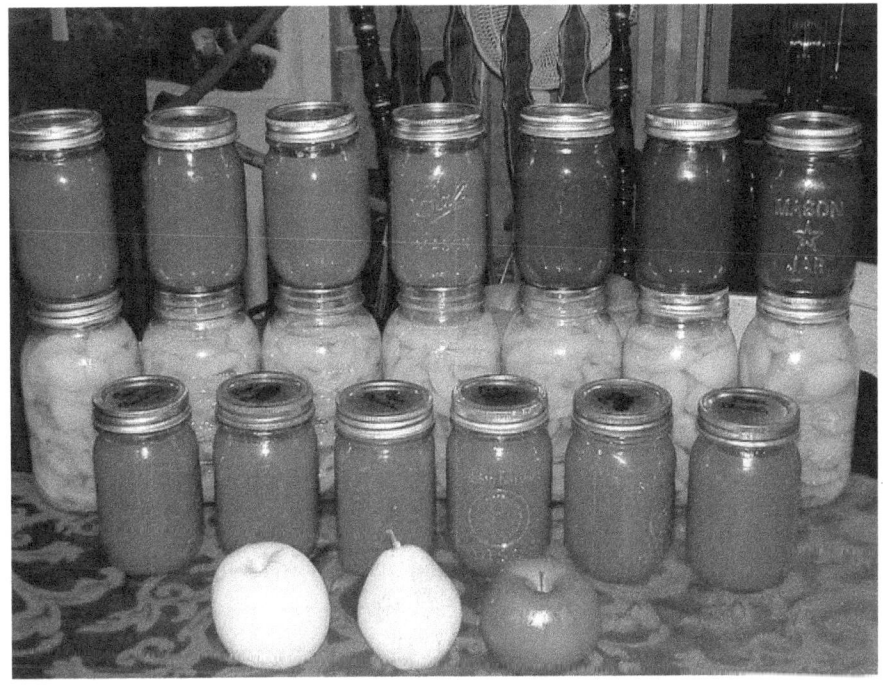

The Prepper's Guide To Food And Water Storage For Disaster Preparedness

By Jim Jackson

Disclaimer

This book is intended to be a general guide, to raise awareness, and to help people make informed decisions in the context of their own personal circumstance.

The author accepts no responsibility for any loss or injury be it personal or financial, as a result for the use or misuse of the information in this book. If you have any doubts or concerns after reading this book, please speak to a qualified person before taking any actions

Contents
Introduction

Chapter 1
Planning Short, Medium & Long Term

Chapter 2
How To Efficiently Store Water

Chapter 3
How To Efficiently Store Food

Chapter 4
Preserving Your Fresh Food

Chapter 5
Replenishing Your Food In A Survival Situation

Chapter 6

Additional Tips and Tricks For An Awesome Survival Food Pantry

Conclusion

Introduction

Prepping has become a household word since the late 90s. Prepping means to prepare for any activity, but in this case, prepping or preparations will not be for a joyous event or for a momentous occasion. It will be preparing for the most important challenge for you and your family: preparing for your survival.

But why prep for this at all? Since 1990, a lot of people have wondered if the end of the world is, indeed, at hand. Many feared the year 2000 because no one was really certain what would happen during this period. But of course, as we are all alive and well today, prepping and planning has become more intense for people that are simply looking out for themselves and for the welfare of their families. Gone is the fear of a new century. It has been replaced by actual and terrible events that could really happen.

From doomsday to political chaos to energy and food crises, it is without a doubt we should all think of the possibility of a total lack of control. Once this happens, food, clean water, medicines and various luxury items will replace cash as currency. Stocking up on food that will last for months is the key to surviving a serious catastrophe. You also need to have a supply of clean drinking water. You also have to prepare for the food supply system to be completely interrupted for months or possibly years. You need to plan ahead for replenishing your food supply with your own garden as well as learning how to hunt and raise animals for food.

Before we get into the planning and stocking portion of your food pantry, it is important to clarify a few rules about survival. Trained survivalists tend to follow the Law of 3s. These laws govern how you go about prioritizing your needs in a survival situation. Because we are focusing on food and water, we will just focus on those laws.

> *You can live 3 days without water.*
> *You can live 3 weeks without food.*

Although you can technically live 3 days without water, that second day is going to be rough. You will already be well on your way to dehydration and suffering some dangerous side effects. Going 3 weeks without food is unpleasant and you will be miserable. After a few days without food, you will be zapped of energy. Your muscles will struggle to move and you may find yourself unable to go out and look for food. This is why most preppers diligently work at building up a survival pantry. If you can prevent dehydration and starvation, why wouldn't you?

Chapter 1

Planning Short, Medium & Long Term

A survival pantry is a place where you stock up on food, water and other important supplies for survival. It is a SEPARATE, UPDATED, VENTILATED and PROTECTED pantry or enclosure. There are many places in your home that you can use as a survival pantry. Ideally, this pantry should be somewhere close to where you plan on holing up in the aftermath of a crisis.

There are four characteristics of every survival pantry that you will want to consider when you are trying to find the right space.

*SEPARATE from your daily pantry or supplies. You don't want to rely on your survival food pantry for your daily food needs. Your survival pantry should be left alone for the most part except when items are getting close to expiring or you are in need. What many people don't realize is the fact that a healthy food storage is a great safety net in case you fall on hard times. You never know when you may lose your job or when a family member will become sick and medical bills make it tough for you to afford food.

*EASILY UPDATED/ROTATED is important. You don't want to choose a place that is difficult to reach. You need to be able to rotate your stock and check for any signs of spoilage. Canned food will typically last for years, but there are times it will spoil. You don't want that sitting in your survival food pantry. It can become a bit of a toxic mess. When you add new items, you need to be able to put them in the back or behind your existing items. If your pantry doesn't allow for this, you will be inclined to slack on your rotation duties.

*VENTILATION** is crucial. While basements and root cellars make excellent pantries, if they are not properly ventilated and there isn't some kind of temperature control, you risk losing all of your food. When you read labels that indicate food has a shelf life of 20 years or 5 years, those times are based on the food being stored in ideal locations. Ventilation is important to keeping down mold growth. You certainly don't want to risk your food supplies being destroyed by toxic mold. Your storage area should be:

- Ventilated
- No extreme heat — above 80 degrees Fahrenheit
- No extreme cold — below 50 degrees Fahrenheit
- No dampness
- Out of direct sunlight

*PROTECTED** from would-be looters. You don't want to advertise your pantry. There are going to be plenty of people, likely some of your neighbors, who didn't take the time to plan and store. The people you considered friendly will become the people you have to protect your supplies from. Keep the majority of your food storage out of sight. In a basement, a closed room or even go so far as to create a false wall in a large room to hide your supplies behind it. You also need to protect your pantry from pesky invaders like mice, ants and roaches. It is extremely frustrating to discover all of your hard work stocking up on food has been destroyed by an infestation.

Do your best to meet each of these requirements. You don't have to have an underground bunker or a safe room in order to have a survival pantry that will keep you and your family alive in the aftermath of a catastrophic event. These characteristics are what you aim for, but a prepper knows, you do the best you can with what you have.

Short, Medium and Long Term Planning

Rome wasn't built in a day and your survival food pantry will not be, either. It doesn't make sense to go into debt trying to stock up on food. You need to do your planning in bite sized pieces. For this reason, you are going to ease into short, medium and, ultimately, long-term planning for your food storage.

Short term is going to be your first milestone. This will be enough food and water to last your family 30 days to 3 months. Expect it to take you at least that long to build up to that amount of food.

Medium term is about 3 to 6 months of food and water on hand. This is where things start to get tricky if you haven't identified a good space for your survival pantry. If you don't have a single space available, you may have to get creative with where you store your food and water.

Long term would be classified as a survival food cache that would last your family for a year or more. This will take a long time to build up to and it will take up a great deal of space. While this is a goal many preppers have, it is something that takes time and dedication to achieve.

Planning Your Pantry-Food

The following tips will help you plan what you need to include in your pantry. Be prepared; you are going to need to do some math here. It is important to point out that storing food for a survival situation is based on calories, not quantity. Today, we tend to eat three meals a day with some snacking in between. Unless you are on a strict diet, you probably don't pay much attention to your calorie intake. It is all about eating until you satisfy your hunger. In a survival situation, you may not get the chance to eat 3 square meals a day. You may only get to eat a single meal with a couple of snacks in between. If you eat the right meal, you can still survival and thrive.

Let's start with a very basic formula that will help you plan out your pantry.

For survival, assume each member of your family needs 2,000 calories per day to survive. Technically, children would need less, but it doesn't hurt to have a little extra food on hand. Men can survive on 2,000 calories per day, but if they are going to be doing any kind of labor-intensive work, i.e. hunting, splitting wood or digging, it would be best if they had an extra 500 to 1000 calories per day.

Let's assume you have a family of 4.4 people x 2000 calories = 8,000 calories per day.

You need to store enough food that will ensure each member of your family is getting their daily calorie requirement. You need to read labels. Canned foods and freeze-dried foods are a favorite among preppers. They store for years without spoiling. Let's say you are going to do the bulk of your prepping with freeze-dried foods (which is an excellent choice if you can afford the high prices).

A #10 can of freeze-dried food will typically hold 16 servings. Don't be fooled into think 16 servings will feed a family of 4, 4 meals. It won't. You need to look at the calorie content on the can.

We need to make another assumption: Let's assume each serving of whatever freeze-dried meal you are serving the family has 250 calories. This is actually pretty standard for freeze-dried and canned foods.

Each family member needs 2000 calories a day. 2000 calories per day/250 calories per serving = 8 meals needed per person to reach daily calorie intake.

Each can holds 16 servings. 16 servings per can divided by 8 meals per person = 2. 2 people will need a single can of food each day. For a family of 4, you would need 2 cans of food per day.

If you are working towards a 30-day food supply, you would need 60 cans of freeze-dried food.

Wowza! To calculate how much food you would need for 60 days, 90 days or however long, use the same formula. Now, obviously you wouldn't want to feed your family the same meal all day, every single day, but this example gives you a better idea of how much food you need to start stocking in your survival food pantry.

Nutrition is just as important (if not more so) in a survival situation as it would be any other typical day. You need to do your best to provide somewhat balanced meals. Look at a food pyramid and try and create a food pantry that will allow you to feed your family diversified yet nutritional meals. We will get into what foods you will want to store to feed your family nutritious meals in another chapter.

Planning Your Pantry - Water

Water is by far the most challenging aspect of a survival food pantry. It is big and bulky and you need a lot of it! How much do you need?

Every member of the family needs 1 gallon of water per day.

If you have just done the math in your head, you know that we are talking about 120 gallons of water for a family of four for a single month. That is a lot of space. Sadly, 120 gallons is only going to provide enough water for drinking and some very basic cleaning and food prep. It isn't enough water to take a bath or do any serious housecleaning.

Despite the challenges of storing water, you still have to do it. You have to come up with a way to keep enough water on hand to keep your family alive. In the following chapter, we will discuss some ways to go about doing that. Before we get to that part though, there is yet another rule of survival.

All water is dirty and unsafe to drink.

If the water is commercially bottled and has been stored in BPA-free containers in prime conditions, you can assume the water is safe to drink. However, that is typically the only time you want to drink water without purifying it.

There are too many life-threatening viruses and bacteria that can be hiding in water that hasn't been treated. It is too risky to even try. Because of this, you will want to keep a supply of water purification methods on hand in your survival pantry. If you have the means, you can boil the water as well. Household bleach is a common method of purifying water, but it only has a shelf life of about 6 months. If you are planning on using bleach to purify your water, it is important you keep a close eye on your rotation. Iodine is also an option, but keep in mind; anybody with an allergy to shellfish will likely be allergic to iodine.

Filters are an option, but they are not purifiers. Meaning, they cannot remove viruses. You can certainly opt to purify water and then filter to make it taste better while making it clearer.

When you are building up your survival food pantry, ask yourself this question: will you be bugging in or bugging out? If you plan on moving to another more secure location, don't waste your time building up a medium or long-term food pantry in your existing home. Hauling all your food and water from Point A to Point B will be extremely difficult and likely impossible. You will need to keep a minimum of 3 days worth of food and water in your home, even if you plan on bugging out. However, it would be a good idea to err on the side of caution and plan a 30-day supply just in case it isn't safe for you to leave immediately following whatever event has befallen you.

Chapter 2

How To Efficiently Store Water

Let's talk water storage. It is a daunting task, but you have to do it. How and where you store water will depend a great deal on where you live or where you plan on holing up after a disaster. Ideally, the goal for most is to be somewhere that is rural. You will need land and space in order to truly thrive when you are dealing with a catastrophic event that has upset the way the country or world operates.

You must assume that the power grid will be down. No power means public water systems are going to fail. They will not be purified, which makes the water coming out of the tap unsafe to drink.

Private Wells

If you have your own well, you will need a hand pump to get the water out. Your electric well pump will be unusable. There are solar pumps out there if you are willing to make the investment. You cannot assume the water that comes out of your well is safe 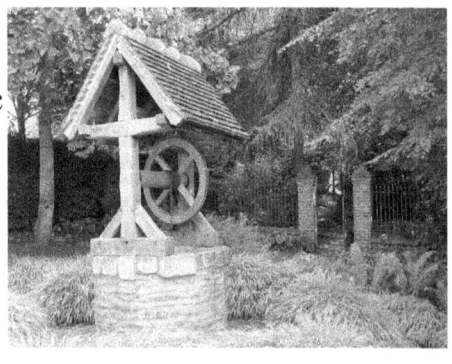 to drink. You just never know what may have happened upriver. There could be dead animals contaminating the water, or a chemical leakage. Always purify the water before drinking it.

Cisterns

These are awesome if you
have the space. The giant
vessels are placed up on a hill
or buried in the ground (which
is great if you want to hide
your water supply). There are
varying sizes of cisterns
ranging from 500-gallon
containers all the way up to
1000 gallons. You will need a
hand pump to get the water
out of the cistern if it is buried.
When it is placed on a hill,
you can take advantage of
gravity.

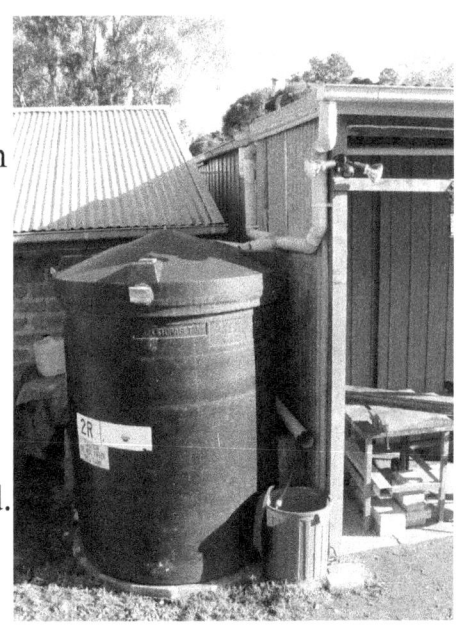

Bottled Water

While bottled water seems
quick and easy, it can get
rather expensive and take up a
lot of room. It would be a
good idea to have a supply of
bottled water on hand for
those times you need a drink,
but don't have the time to go
through the purification
process. You are probably
thinking, "Hey, I will just use
those milk jugs and bottle my
own water." In theory, you
would be on to something.

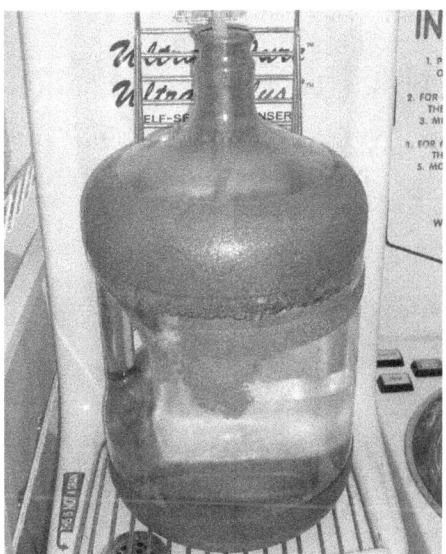

However, you do not want to use old milk jugs. They will break down in a matter of months and leak everywhere. You can use old juice bottles, 2-liter soda bottles and old water bottles. Wash the bottles with soap and water and refill with water from your tap. Some people will add a drop or two of bleach to the water to preserve it. Most tap water is already treated with some chlorine. You don't absolutely need to add the additional bleach, but it won't hurt if you do. You will want to cycle your home-bottled water out every 6 months or so. Use the water to water the garden, rinse and refill.

Rain Barrels

This is an excellent option and it is virtually free. You can make your own rain barrel for about $10 or buy one at Home Depot. Fill as many barrels as you can with the rainwater that runs off your roof. Now, rainwater is generally 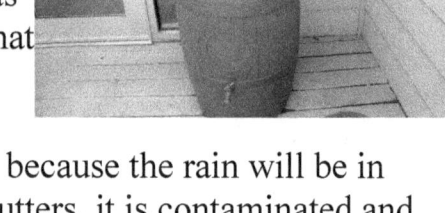 considered safe to drink, but because the rain will be in contact with your roof and gutters, it is contaminated and will need to be purified before drinking.

Backyard Ponds

Yes, you can drink pond water if you purify it. It doesn't take much to dig a pond. You can have a small pond that is lined with plastic or a large pond that is au natural, meaning it has a rocky, dirt floor. For an added bonus, add some fish to the pond for a renewable food source. If your pond is murky, fill your vessel with the water 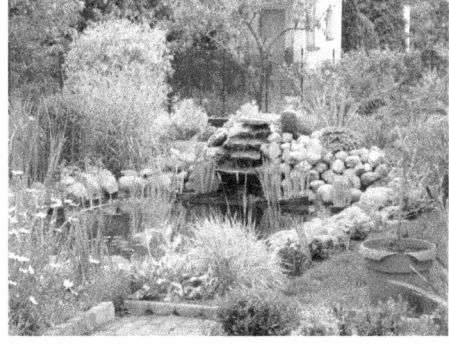 that is between the green layer on top and the dirt on the bottom. It helps to filter your pond water before purifying it.

Swimming Pools/Hot Tubs

If you have one or both of these recreational items, you have an excellent water supply on hand. You will want to wait to purify the water from the pool or hot tub for at least three days following the power going out. This gives the chlorine time to evaporate 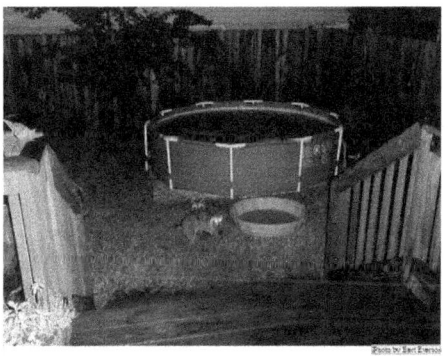 a bit to bring it down to a safe level for consumption. Rain will help replenish the water.

Chapter 3

How To Efficiently Store Food

Storing food is so important. You need to make sure you maximize space and get the longest shelf-life possible out of your food. You need to plan on living without power, which means you will not have refrigeration available. You won't be able to reach into the freezer and pull out steaks for dinner. You are relegated to either finding fresh meat or living off of canned, dehydrated or freeze-dried meat. It is time to talk about the storage of all that food you are going to be stocking up on for your survival food pantry.

Shelving

Now that you have a fairly good idea about the amount of food you are going to need to start stocking up on, you need to figure out how you are going to store it. A simple rule of thumb is to keep your food at least 6 inches off the ground. This will keep your food safe and dry in the event there is MINOR flooding.

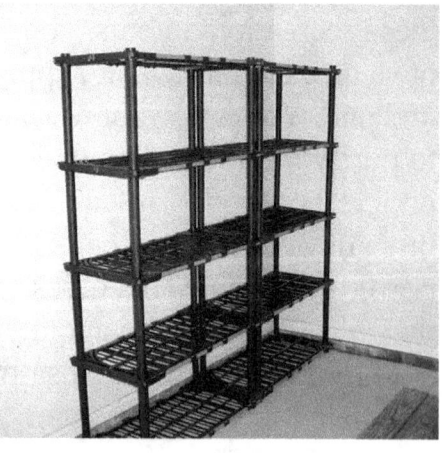

Please know that 6 inches isn't all that much, but if the washing machine in the basement goes crazy one day or you have a pipe burst, your food should be A-OK.

Choose shelves that have a lip in front to keep food from

sliding forward and off. If you live in an area prone to earthquakes or close to train tracks that may cause enough vibration for the food to slide forward, this is especially important. If you are holing up and riding out a storm with your food pantry, you don't want a falling can of chili to land on your head. If the shelf doesn't have a lip, there are plenty of shelves you can put together upside down to get the necessary lip. It works!

You can also use rope tied tight across the front of the shelving, about 3 inches up, to keep your food in place. A piece of wood across the front would also work. It is all about getting creative to keep your food secure.

Food-Grade Buckets

Food-grade 5-gallon buckets are a prepper's best friend. You can't live without them. They are your best bet to keeping your food fresh and safe from pests. They are also a lot easier to stack and will keep your food from spilling all over if there is some kind of event that causes shelves to fall or move. Check with restaurants and bakeries to see if you can either have or buy their old buckets. You will be surprised at how many restaurants are willing to give these things away. One man's trash is most certainly another man's

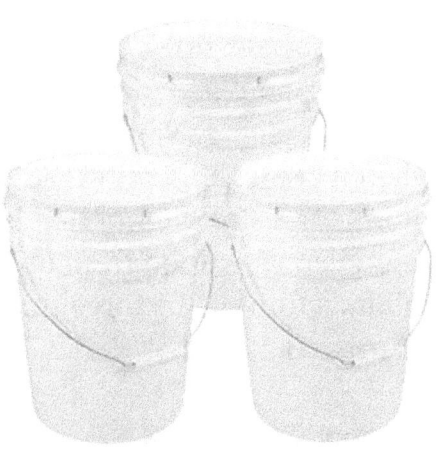

treasure. The buckets need lids. Don't bother if they don't have the lids. Do not use buckets that have held chemicals or fertilizers.

Mylar Bags

These bad boys are another favorite among preppers. Contrary to popular belief, they do not keep out mice. However, they will keep out pests like ants and cockroaches. Ideally, you will want to put your dried grains and beans into the Mylar bag, 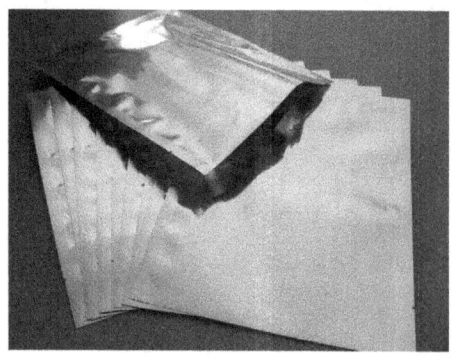 seal it and then place it in a 5-gallon bucket. When stored like this, you can extend the shelf-lives of some items to 20 years or more! Do yourself a favor and buy the bags in bulk. You will use them. You can even store boxes of pasta inside the bags and place them on your shelf. Just make sure you label everything. You have a couple of different options when it comes to sealing the bag. Most are heat-sealed with an iron or a special tool that is basically a Foodsaver. The bags keep your food from being exposed to light, oxygen and moisture — the three things that shorten shelf-lives and destroy your food.

Kitchen Necessities

You are going to have to learn to cook without all of your fancy appliances. Take a look at your kitchen right now. How do you open your canned food or heat up your chili? You probably have an electric can opener, microwave and even a coffee maker to make your life easier. It's time to go back to the Dark Ages — so to speak.

The following is a list of tools you will want to have on hand in your survival food pantry.

- Manual can opener
- Manual grain mill
- Solar stove — you can build or buy one
- Percolated coffee pot
- Manual hand mixer
- Dutch oven
- Cast iron cookware — ideal for cooking over an open fire
- Sterno stove
- Coleman stove — store plenty of fuel/propane tanks
- Hand-cranked food strainer
- Heavy-duty hot pads
- Hand-cranked blender

What to Store

This is what you have been waiting for, right? What should you be storing in your survival pantry? Are you ready for another survival rule?

Only store what you eat today.

If you and your family loathe carrots, don't bother wasting your time and money stocking up on canned or freeze-dried carrots. Your taste buds are not suddenly going to change because the world went to heck in a handbasket. Of course if you were absolutely starving, you would probably eat the carrots, but you are building up a survival pantry so you won't have to worry about starving. You don't need the stress of trying to convince your kids to eat the carrots. Give them what they eat today and your life will be much easier for it. Survival is stressful enough without worrying about picky eaters.

We are going to break this down into food groups. You should pick and choose what you and your family eats and stock up on it. It is important you diversify your meals. There is such a thing as food fatigue. If you eat canned chili every day for a month, your body is going to rebel. You will suffer severe intestinal upset that could put you at risk of dehydration. Change things up a bit to keep your body happy. This list is a combination of freeze-dried, dried, canned and standard grocery items.

Grains
- Wheat
- Flour
- Cornmeal
- Oats
- Rice

Legumes/Beans
- Pinto beans
- Navy beans
- Kidney beans

- Black beans — excellent for making patties for burgers!

Fruit
- Canned fruits — whatever your family likes
- Dehydrated fruits — great snacks as is
- Freeze-dried fruits — eat as is or reconstitute to give a more "normal" taste

Vegetables
- Canned veggies — whatever your family likes; choose low-sodium varieties when possible
- Dehydrated veggies
- Freeze-dried veggies — toss in with rice to make a hearty stew

Protein/Meat
- Tuna
- Salmon
- Spam
- Chicken
- Peanut butter — it is high in protein
- Jerky

Dairy
- Powdered butter
- Powdered eggs
- Instant milk — best for drinking
- Powdered milk — best for cooking
- Powdered cheese

Spices

- Salt
- Pepper
- Garlic salt and powder
- Bay leaves
- All-seasoning

Baking

- Baking soda
- Baking powder
- Cooking oil
- Shortening
- Yeast — short shelf-life can make this a problem

Grocery Store Items

- Pasta
- Crackers
- Granola
- Candy
- Chocolate
- Sugar
- Honey
- Coffee
- Tea
- Nuts
- Chocolate bars
- Chili, ravioli, Spaghettios, etc…
- Canned beans
- Tomato sauce
- Macaroni and Cheese

- Drink mixes — go for the kind that do not require you to add sugar

This list is not all-inclusive. Your best bet is to take a look at your pantry right now. What food do you have in there? That is the food you want to start stocking up on. You will be preparing your meals from scratch so you need to make sure you have everything on hand to do so.

It helps to write down your family's favorite meals. What recipes do you use most often? If you are one of those really organized people who makes weekly or monthly meal plans, take a look at your plan and calculate the ingredients you use in a recipe. Multiply the ingredients by 12, assuming you would make that one meal once a month for a year. This will help give you an idea of how much food to stock in your food pantry.

Example: Rice and Veggies
To feed your family, you use 2 cups of rice and one can of mixed vegetables. Multiply the rice by 12 (2 cups x 12 = 24 cups of rice for a year). One can of veggies x 12 = 12 cans for the year. A single pound of rice is equal to about 2 cups. You would need 12 pounds of rice to last your family a year if you only used it to cook that one meal, once a month.

While that is one way to go about figuring how much to store, you can skip the math and just use rough estimates. The idea behind that example is to show you just how much food it takes to feed your family a single meal. It can be hard to fathom when you have 20 grocery stores to run to when you need a particular ingredient to make a meal. In a survival situation, whatever is in your pantry is all you have.

Don't skimp on the little luxuries like chocolate, coffee and candy. They may not be crucial to your survival, but they do help you feel normal. Surviving something catastrophic is as much mental as it is physical. You want to feel somewhat normal and you want your kids to feel normal. Living every minute on edge and terrified isn't going to do you any good. If you can wake up and enjoy your cup of coffee as you plan your day of chopping wood, hauling water or skinning the animal you caught in your snare, it helps give you a more positive outlook.

Chapter 4

Preserving Your Fresh Food

You can save a ton of money and gain a valuable skill by learning how to preserve the food you grow, harvest from the wild or buy in bulk. You don't have to buy canned food at the grocery store. Canning food in your own kitchen gives you the luxury of picking the best fruits and vegetables to feed your family while keeping out preservatives.

You will want to start growing your own garden today to brush up on your skills for the future. In the event of a long-term crisis, you are going to have to grow your own food. There is a learning curve to gardening and it is best to figure it out today while you have the luxury of running to the grocery store when needed.

Canning

Canning fruits and vegetables is fairly simple. Anybody can do it with the right equipment. You can watch videos online, read books or take a class through your local college about how to safely can food. There are some basic supplies you will need to get started canning.

- Pressure Canner
- Mason jars
- Bands and lids
- Canning tongs
- Funnel

- Strainer
- Pectin — for jams
- Vinegar and pickling spices for pickling
- Canning salt

Visit your local farmer's market or local farms that offer the best deals on bulk fruits and vegetables. Choose organic whenever possible. It is a little more costly, but the flavor is better and you won't have to worry about pesticides and herbicides.

Always make sure you sterilize your jars, lids and bands before canning. Failure to do so could result in contamination and all of your hard work will be for naught. Bacteria within the sealed jar will cause food spoilage. Most extension offices and the CDC will recommend you only store home-canned food for 6 months to a year, but if you do it right and store it properly you can extend the shelf-life for several years.

You don't have to limit your canning to fruits, veggies and meat. You can create soup and stew mixes that are ready to go with just a little water to rehydrate the food. Imagine homemade chicken soup in a jar! You will need to spend some time researching various recipes and learning the tricks to preserving food, but it is well worth it.

Dehydrating
Dehydrating fruits, vegetables, meat and spices is another way to save a lot of money while building up your survival

food pantry. You will need to invest in a good dehydrator. The Excalibur is a favorite among preppers as it does the job and it does it fairly quickly. You can store your dehydrated foods in mason jars or use a Foodsaver to store the food in sealed bags.

Jerky is pretty expensive in the store, but you can certainly make it at home for a fraction of the cost. Experiment with various seasoning recipes to come up with the perfect taste for you and your family.

You can use Mylar bags to store your dehydrated foods. This is an excellent choice as it removes the oxygen from the bag and keeps the food fresher, for longer. Invest in silica packs to toss into your jars or bags with your dehydrated products. If you don't remove as much of the moisture from the food as possible, you risk it molding.

Dehydration involves removing the majority of the water from a food. Unfortunately, the water or juices of a food are where a lot of the nutrients are. Dehydrated food is great for snacking on, but shouldn't be used to fulfill your daily calorie needs. It simply doesn't have all the nutrients you need to stay healthy.

Chapter 5

Replenishing Your Food In A Survival Situation

If disaster strikes before you have built up a long-term food pantry, you need to be prepared to replenish your pantry. If you have endured a minor natural disaster that will interrupt the food supply for a few weeks, you won't need to worry too much about this area. However, do you really know what disaster may befall you? No. And for that reason, you need to prepare for anything.

To replenish your food supply, you need to grow your own food. This includes raising animals to use as a food source. Some of the easiest animals to raise that don't require a lot of space include chickens, rabbits, and pigs. Cows are a little more difficult to raise and are not quite as prolific. You would be better off investing in smaller animals.

Because you never know what kind of travesty will strike, you need to keep a supply of seeds on hand to help start your garden. Don't buy the typical seeds you find in your gardening store. You need to purchase heirloom seeds.

Heirloom seeds are necessary because they are the only kind that will produce vegetables that contain seeds that can be replanted. The typical $1 packs of seeds that are on the market will not produce vegetables with seeds that will produce more plants. You may get the seed to sprout, but there is only a slim chance it will produce any edible vegetables. When you spend the extra money to buy heirloom seeds, you are ensuring you will have a renewable food source for years to come.

Buy in bulk and throw the seeds in the refrigerator for now. When the power fails and the refrigeration is out, store your seeds somewhere cool and dark to keep them from sprouting.

Hunting

Learn how to hunt. Now, today you may have an aversion to shooting Bambi, but when you and your family are hungry, you will be able to take the deer down. You can choose to use a gun or get familiar with a bow and arrow. If you are opting for the gun, stock up on ammunition. You can also learn how to set snares and traps. This is a great way to hunt small game. Don't turn your nose up at the thought of eating squirrels and other animals you trap in the wild. Food is food and with the spices you have stored and are growing, you can dress it up and make it into a tasty meal.

Foraging

It is crucial you learn how to forage, as well. There are hundreds of plants that grow in the wild that are edible and full of various vitamins and minerals. In fact, plants in the wild can also be used medicinally. You will definitely want to buy a couple of books and read up on the subject. You can't go around eating every plant you find. Follow these steps if you are not sure whether or not a plant is safe to eat.

1. Rub a portion of the plant on the inside of your wrist. Wait 15 to 30 minutes and check to see if there is any negative reaction. Redness, itchiness or burning is a sign the plant is toxic and should be avoided. If you don't experience a

reaction, move on to step two.

2. Place a small portion of the plant under your tongue. If it is toxic, you will probably know right away. However, wait 15 to 30 minutes to see if there is a reaction. Burning, swelling of the tongue or a tingling sensation indicates it is toxic. If there is no negative reaction, move on to step three.

3. Eat a portion of the plant. Wait 24 hours to determine if there is any negative reaction. Digestive issues like diarrhea, vomiting or cramping are signs that you don't want to eat the plant. If there is no negative reaction, you can eat the plant in moderation. You don't want to overdo it.

Chapter 6

Additional Tips and Tricks For An Awesome Survival Food Pantry

You can learn a lot talking with other preppers and experienced survivalists. People have been fine-tuning the art of prepping for decades. Learn from other people's mistakes and successes. You don't have to reinvent the wheel.

- When storing food in buckets, add a few bay leaves to the bottom. This helps repel pests.

- When boiling water to purify it, you don't have to boil it for 15 minutes or even 5 minutes. The moment the water hits boiling point, it is purified.

- Don't buy commercial cans of food. You won't have a refrigerator to store the leftovers in. Unless you plan on feeding 10 people for one meal, these big cans are a waste of money and space.

- Buy in bulk whenever possible. However, do the math and make sure you are getting a good deal.

- Use coupons, especially those 'buy one get one free' deals. It is an excellent way to build up your survival food pantry.

- Budget about $50 a month to building up your survival food pantry if you can afford it.

- Invest in a cookbook that contains recipes designed to work in a survival situation.

Conclusion

Don't get too caught up in the idea of filling your pantry with a ton of food. It's a process that is going to take some time. When you next go grocery shopping, grab 2 cans of kidney beans instead of the one you normally buy. This is one way you can add a little at a time to your pantry without cutting too deeply into your monthly food budget.

Taking the time and energy to stock up a food pantry today will give you peace of mind for the future. You won't have to stress about how you are going to feed your family in the coming months. Having a well-stocked pantry frees you up to work on other things that are necessary for survival, like securing shelter and finding a way to keep your family warm. Every little bit you do today will benefit you in the future.

From The Author

Thank you for taking the time to read this book. As an author, I understand the importance of creating books which my readers will find both enjoyable and informative. If you have the time and feel generous, please don't hesitate to leave an honest review of this book..........Jim Jackson

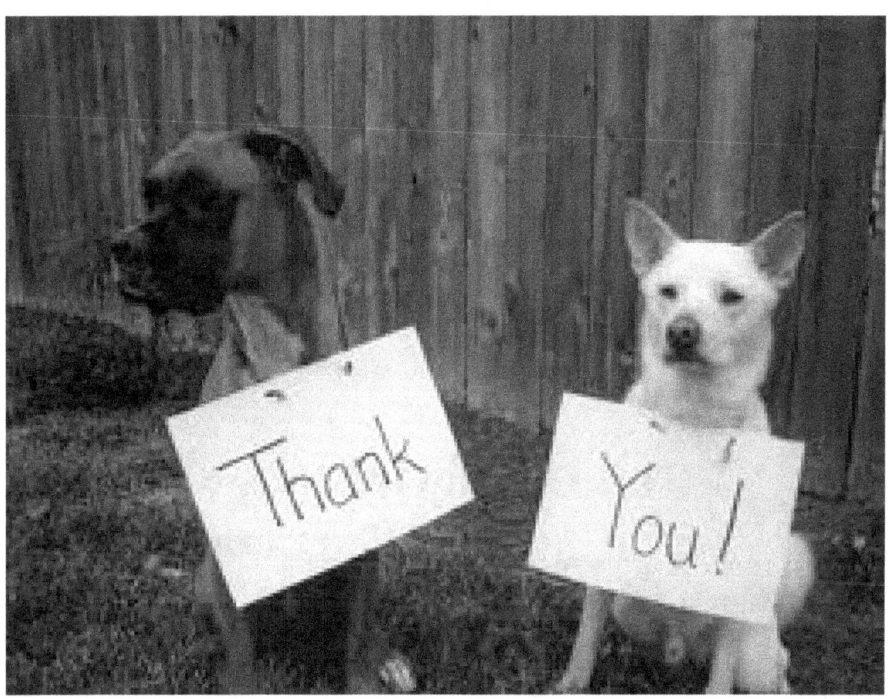

Other Books By Jim Jackson

Camping And Cooking For Beginners

Everyone has a camping disaster story and rarely do they have anything to do with wild animals. From forgetting the food to discovering the tent is too small—a myriad of things can go wrong, but with Camping And Cooking For Beginners, your problems are solved. Beginning with the basics, this handy helper starts with a checklist of what you need for your trip. Choosing the right tent, the right sleeping bag and how to start fires without 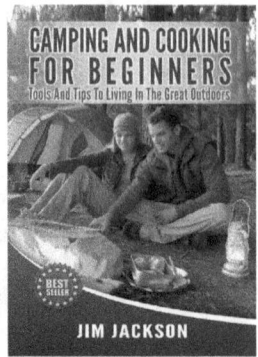 matches (and he's not talking about rubbing two sticks together!) are only a few chapters in the book. The best advice is the authors Top Ten Mistakes First Time Campers Make (and how to avoid them!)—it is invaluable. Get your copy today, before your camping trip and transform your camping experience into the best memory ever!

The Death Of Money

Surviving an economic collapse requires that you be prepared. This small guide will enable you to formulate a plan, allowing you to be proactive instead of reactive to a catastrophic financial crisis. In four chapters, you will gain invaluable knowledge and insight into what it takes to ensure you and your family have the tools necessary to survive the devastating impact of the loss of paper assets. Discover the skills you need to withstand the perils of a vulnerable financial system.

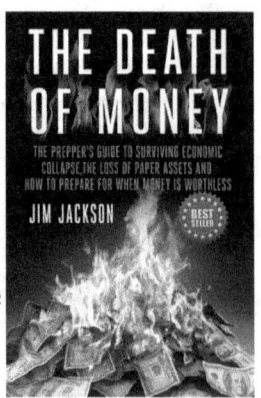

Motorhome Living For Beginners

When you want to change your lifestyle entirely, you need to have enough motivation but you also need to have knowledge about the lifestyle that you are adopting. Many people who want to live in an RV full-time fail to find a balance in their lives which make that living pleasurable, while others can live the dream and learn to compromise on comforts for the sake of freedom. They wake up in the mornings to feel that they have breathed fresh air. They see different scenery every morning

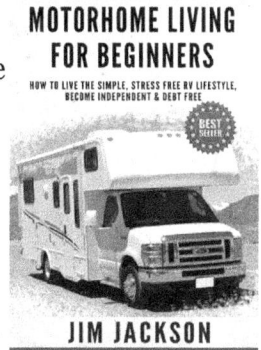

if they so wish. What you need to know before joining them is whether you're cut out for the lifestyle and what differences there are between living in a conventional home and living in an RV. This book bridges that gap in your knowledge, and although you may choose to save a fortune by staying at home, you may also choose the lesser traveled road and discover the benefits of living in an RV.

Both lifestyles, either in an RV or a home, have their pros and cons. Many who choose the RV lifestyle find that adapting their lives comes naturally. It takes a unique and free spirited person to compromise on the luxuries of home living in favor of the adventurous lifestyle offered by RV living, though many do. Once you weigh the pros and cons, you can make the choice wisely, and that's what this book is all about. The book will appeal to the free spirited who seek something more than merely surviving month to month oppressed by mortgage payments and housing taxes.

Both have benefits, though those who live the life they choose, rather than the life chosen for them by responsibility, find that RV life tests their personal boundaries and skills freeing up their lives to live beyond the grid. Journey with us and learn if livingin an RV will suit you, and be prepared for the journey of your life.